MW00910015

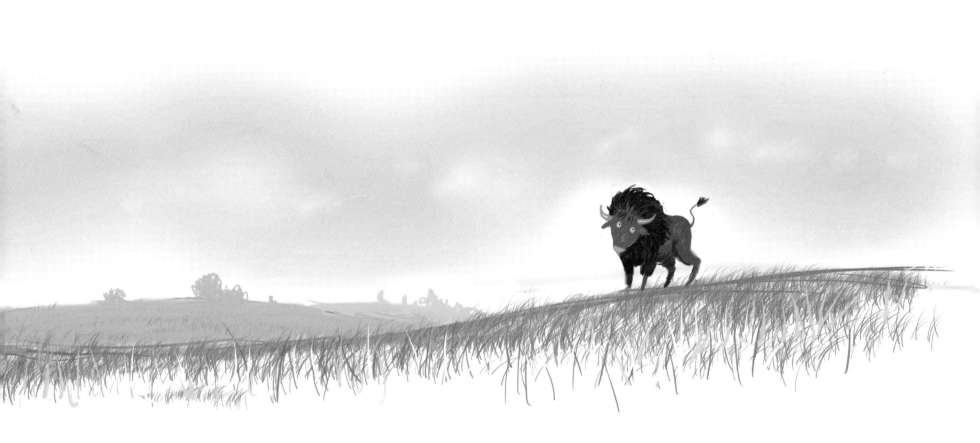

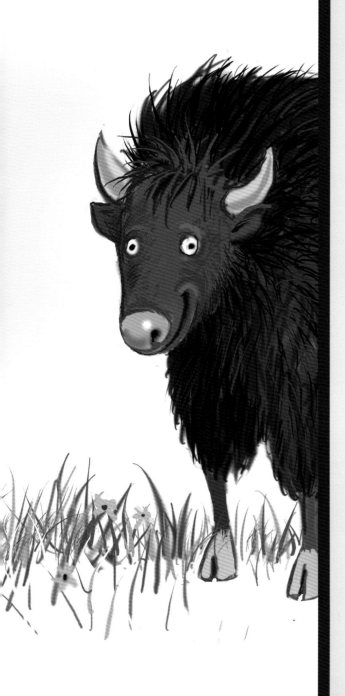

This book belongs to

_____

_____

Written by Wilheimina Long
Illustrated by Ron Miller

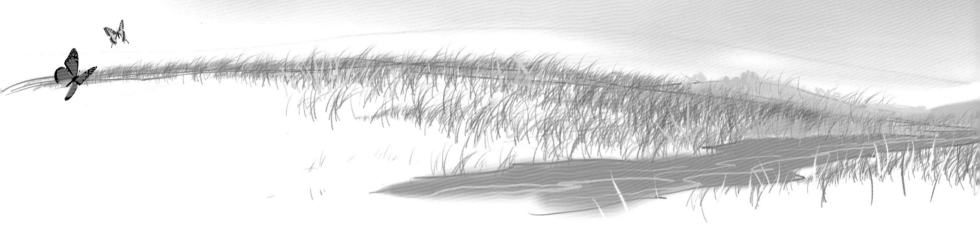

JELLYBEANS
Children's Books

This second edition published by Jellybeans Children's Books Publishing Inc. in June 2013

Text copyright © 2012, 2013 by Wilheimina Long
Illustrations copyright © 2012 by Ron Miller

All rights reserved. No part of this publication may be reproduced or transmitted in any form or by any means, electronic or mechanical, including photocopy, recording, or any information storage and retrieval system, without permission in writing from the publisher.

www.raythebuffalo.com

ISBN: 978-0-9896596-0-4

Printed in China

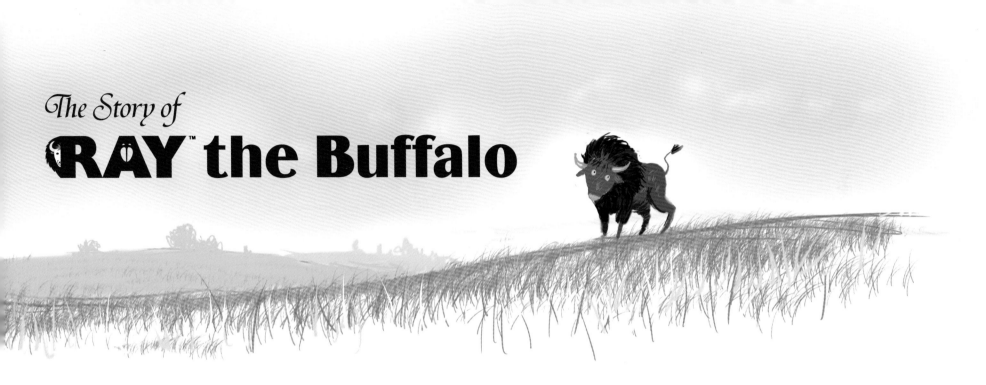

The Story of RAY™ the Buffalo

DEDICATION

This first published edition is dedicated to
my Cousin/God-Daughter SaVanna Noel Jackson and
my Great-Nephew Makhi Aiden Simmons.

Thanks, Ron Miller — my mentor and friend, for having been on my team since 1981, and for being a forever friend — Thanks for the beautiful illustrations that children will enjoy for years to come. Thanks, family and friends, for your expression of support in this endeavor — I am confident that children everywhere will now have two new storybook friends to share their world by way of the book's characters, Ray and Emily.

Emily the Eagle was named in tribute to Second Lieutenant Emily Jazmin Tatum Perez, US Army.

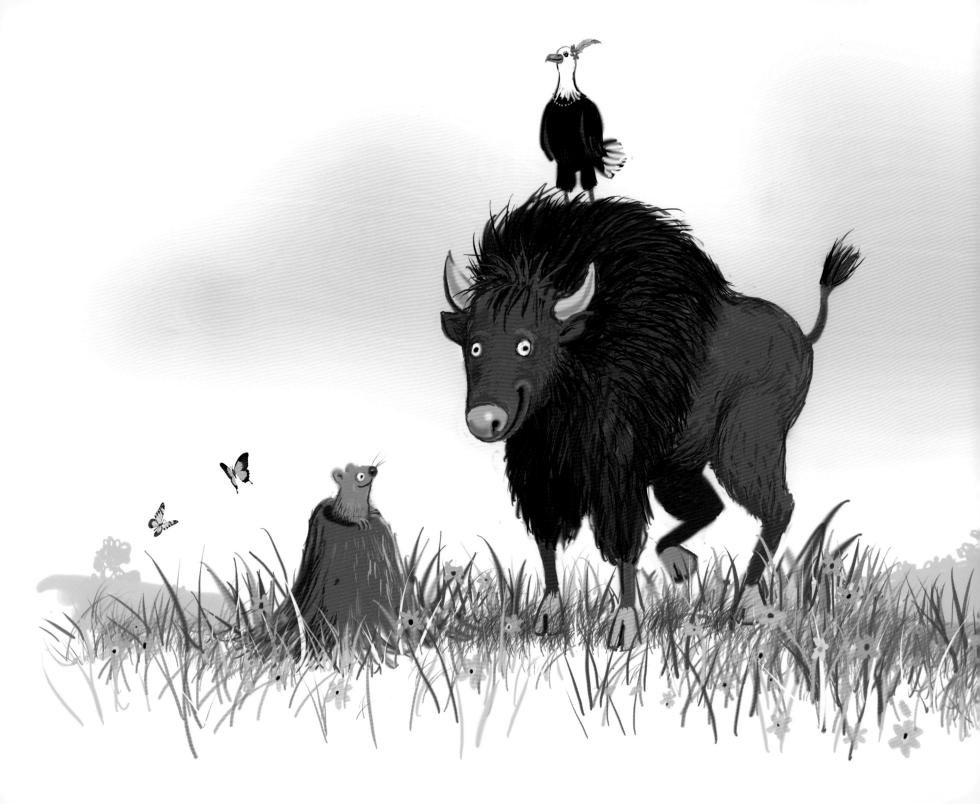

Ray the buffalo is strong and brave like a troop,
even though he belongs to the animal group.

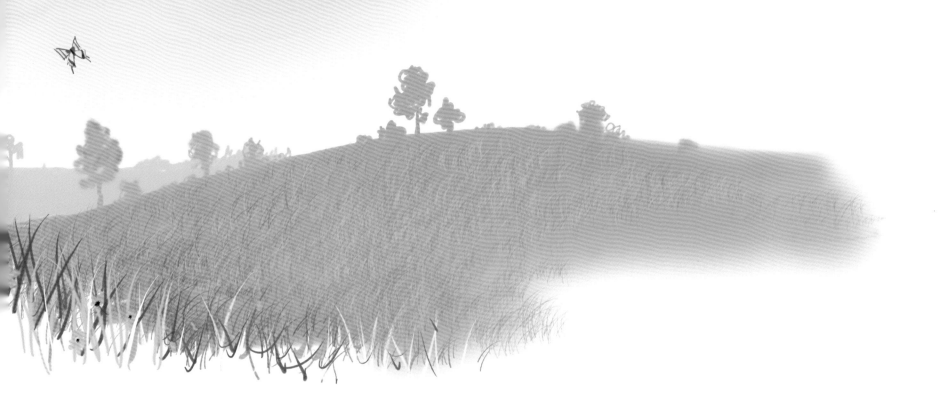

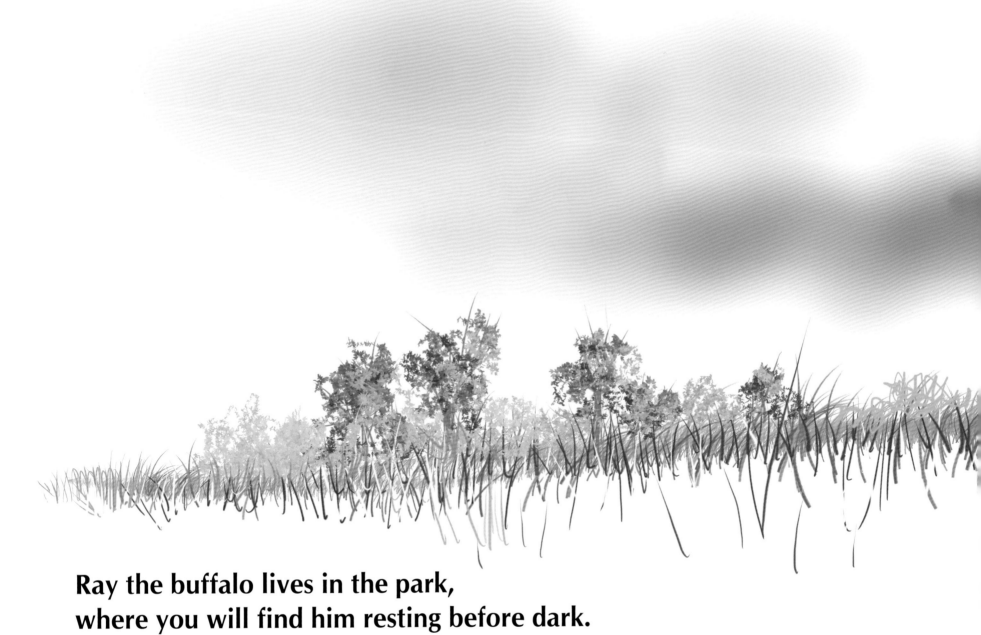

**Ray the buffalo lives in the park,
where you will find him resting before dark.**

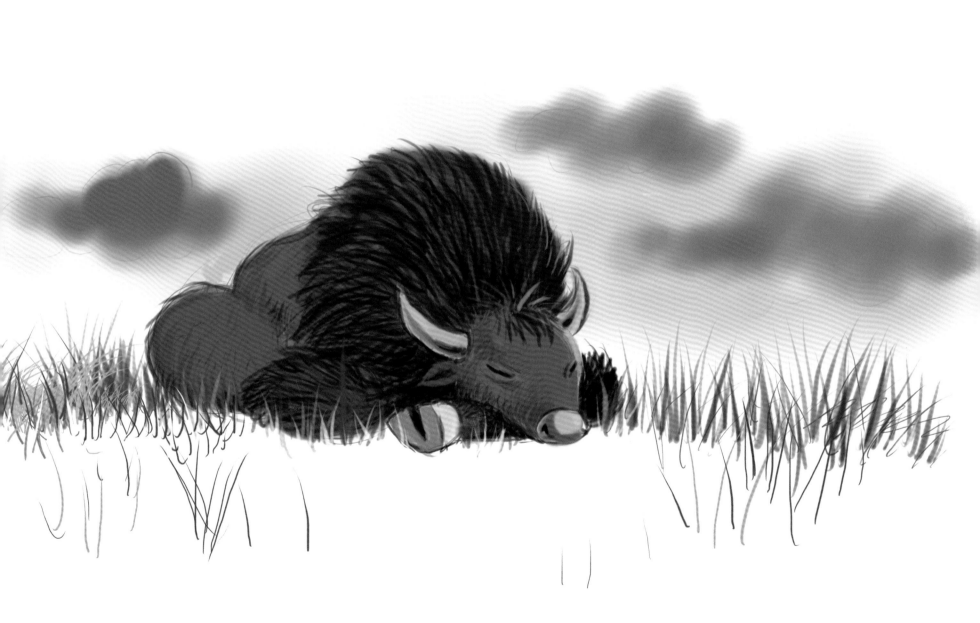

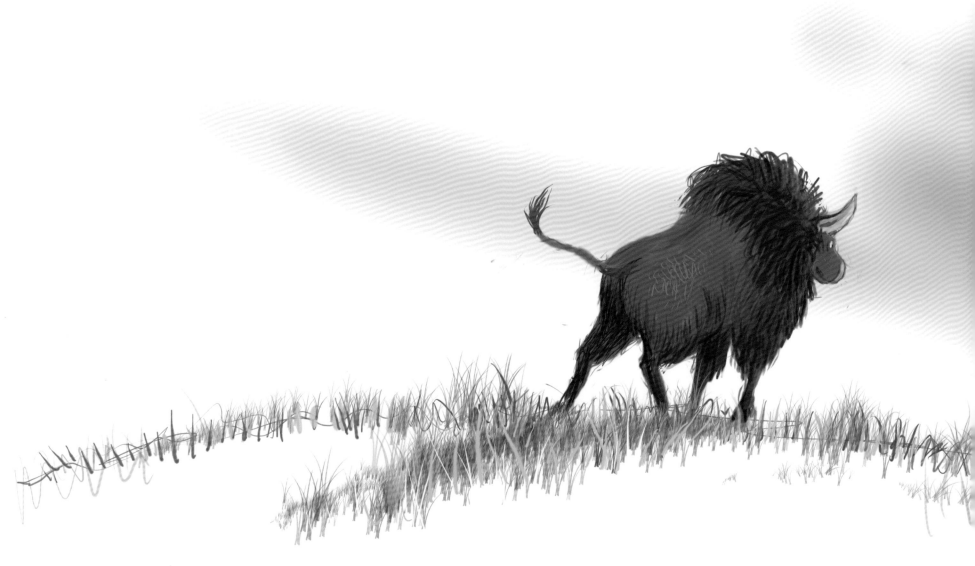

As the sun rises in the east, so does Ray the buffalo.
He stretches and stretches and moves real slow.
But with great pride, he continues his stride.

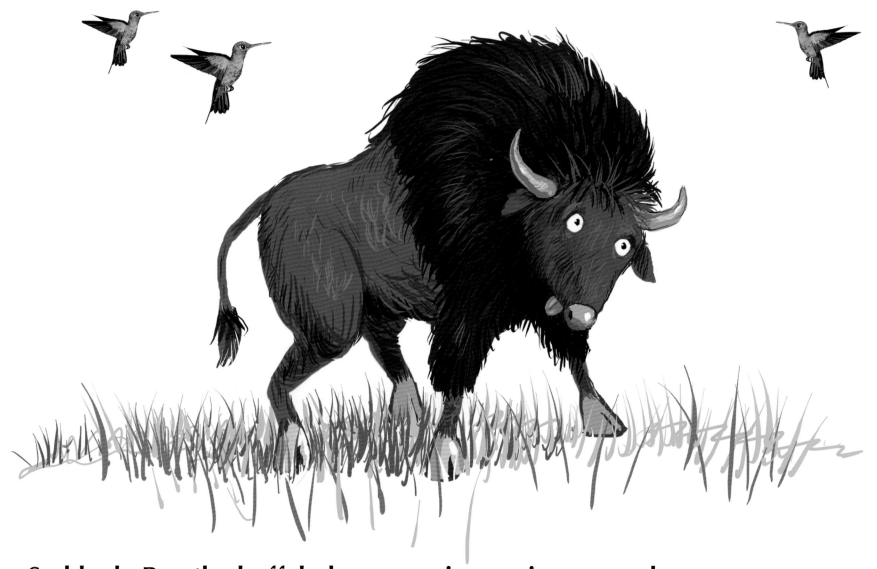

Suddenly Ray the buffalo hears music, music, everywhere.
And he starts to prance and dance, without a care.
But his dancing and prancing does not last.
Ray the buffalo tries real hard, but his prancing is not fast.

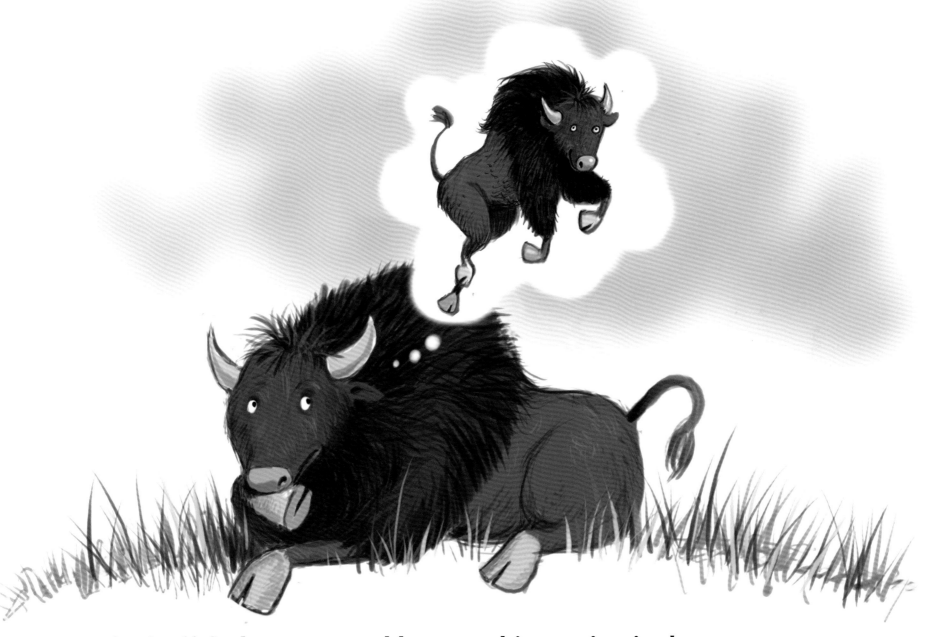

Ray the buffalo becomes sad because his moving is slow.
"Why can't I dance?" he thinks to himself.
"Is it because I'm not very strong?" He does not know.

Above the trees, Ray the buffalo sees Emily the eagle — his friend.
Emily is dancing, dancing, and dancing in the wind.

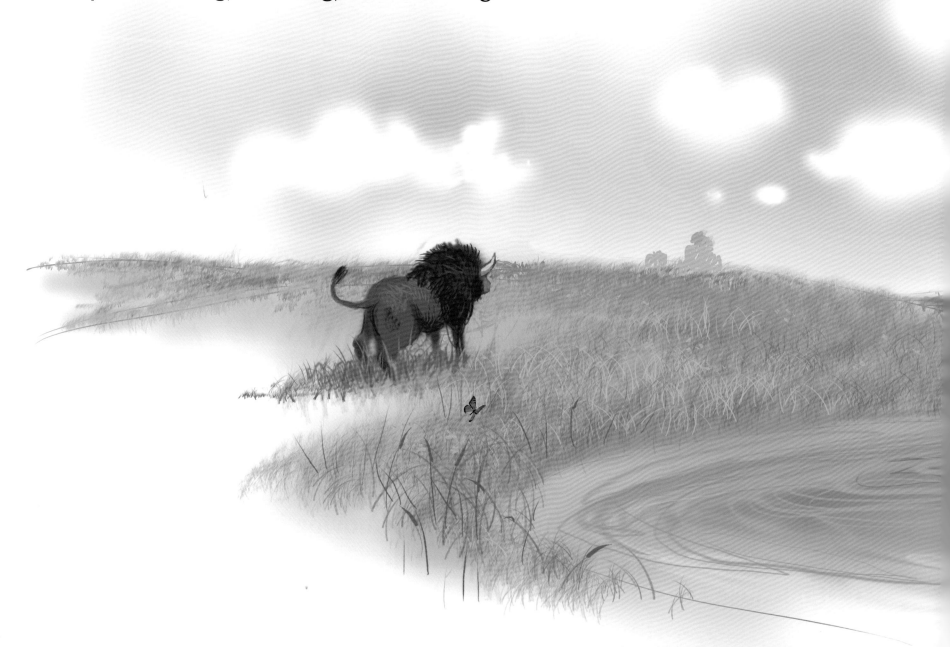

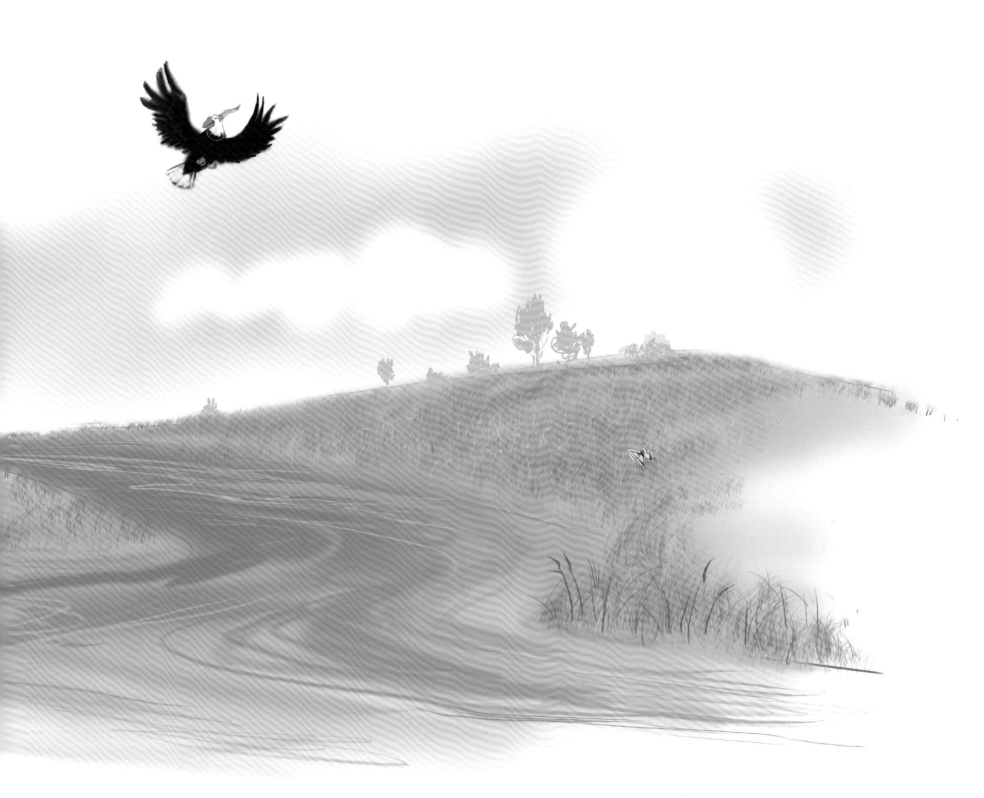

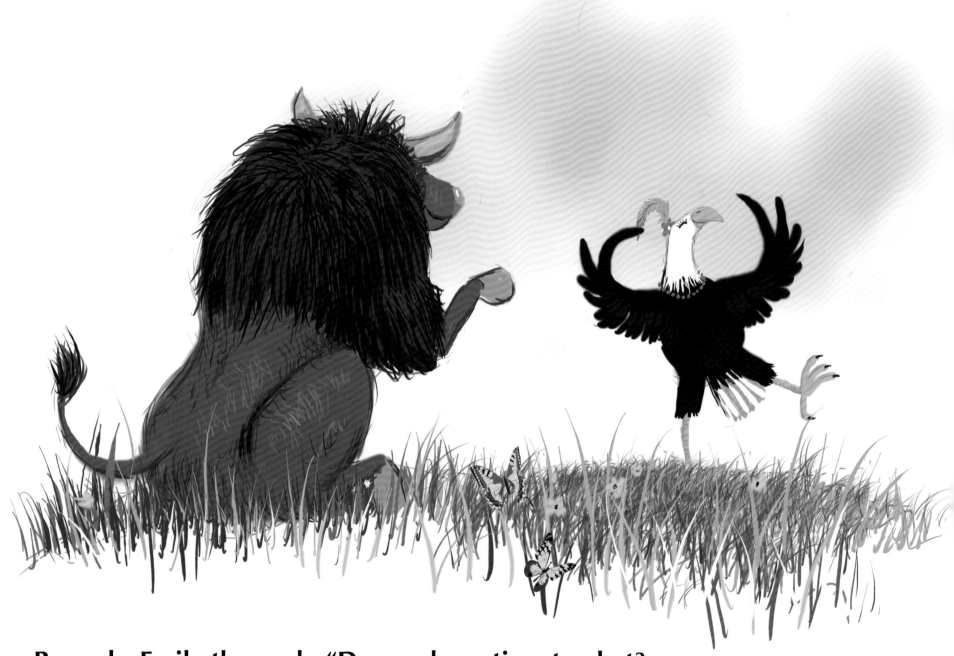

Ray asks Emily the eagle "Do you have time to chat?
And can you tell me how to dance like that?"

"You too can soar like an eagle if you believe," Emily said
"and show off that beautiful brown crown around your head".

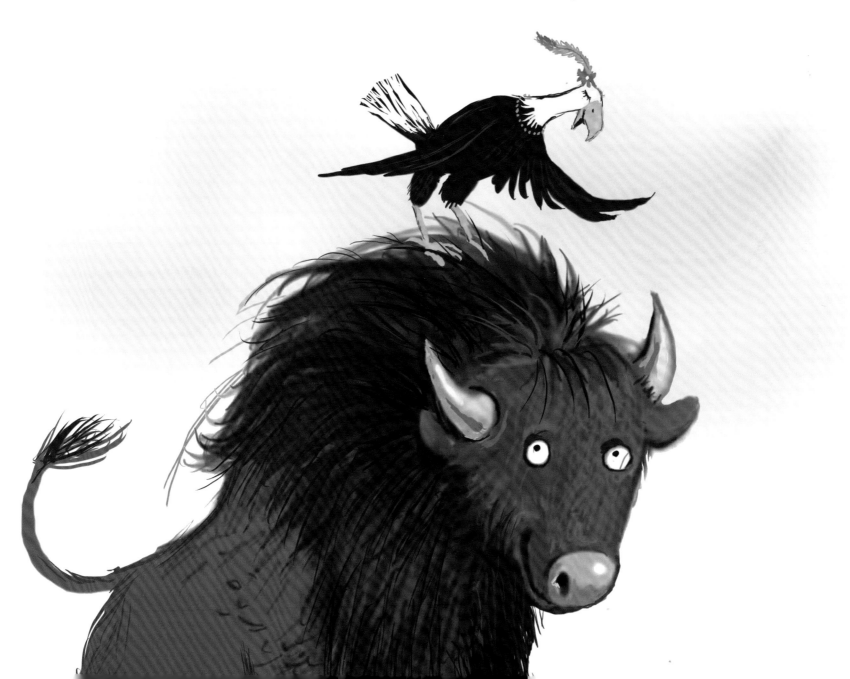

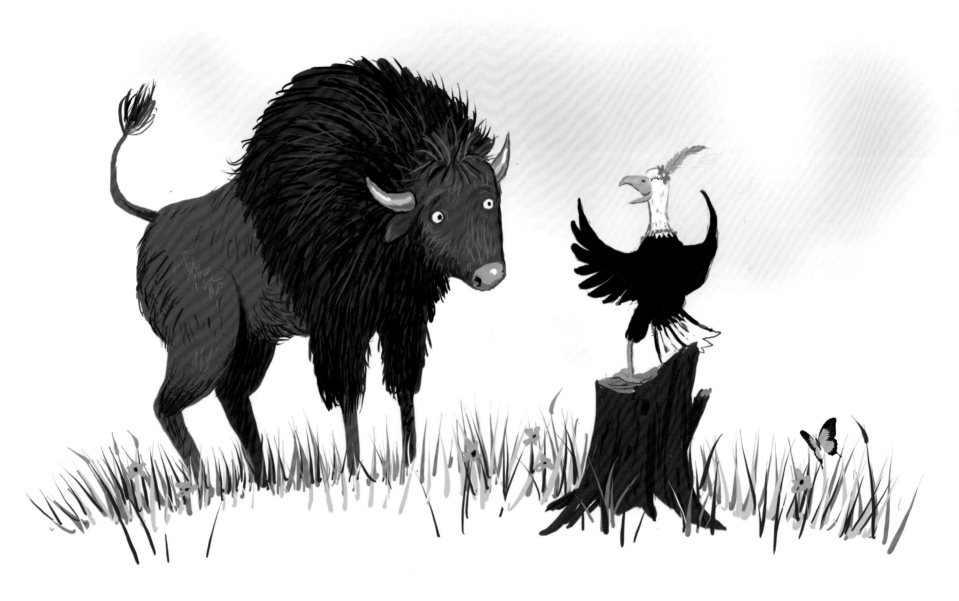

"I am your friend" Emily the eagle replies.
"And I can help you, Ray" she adds, with joy in her eyes.

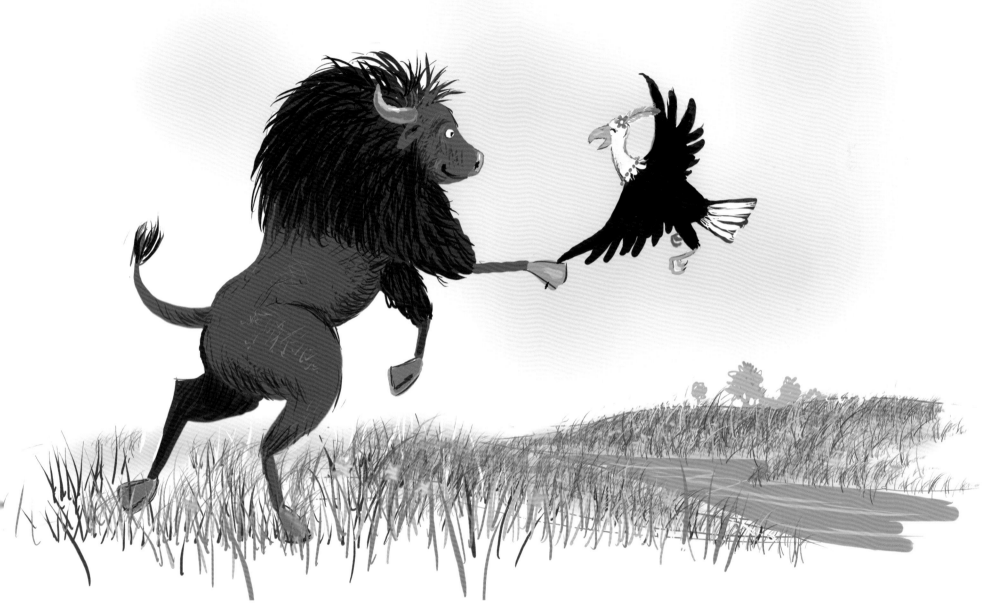

Emily the eagle says "I can show you, Ray.
But you must not sleep all night and all day.
Will you run and play as I lead the way?"

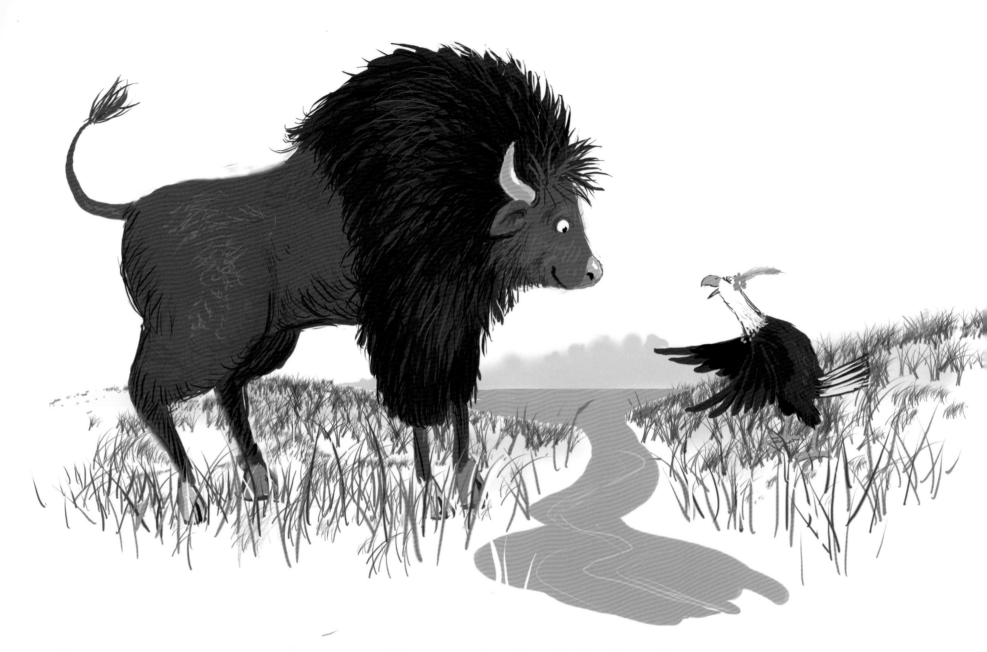

His friend Emily the eagle tells Ray the buffalo that he can't go wrong when he drinks lots of water to stay healthy and strong.

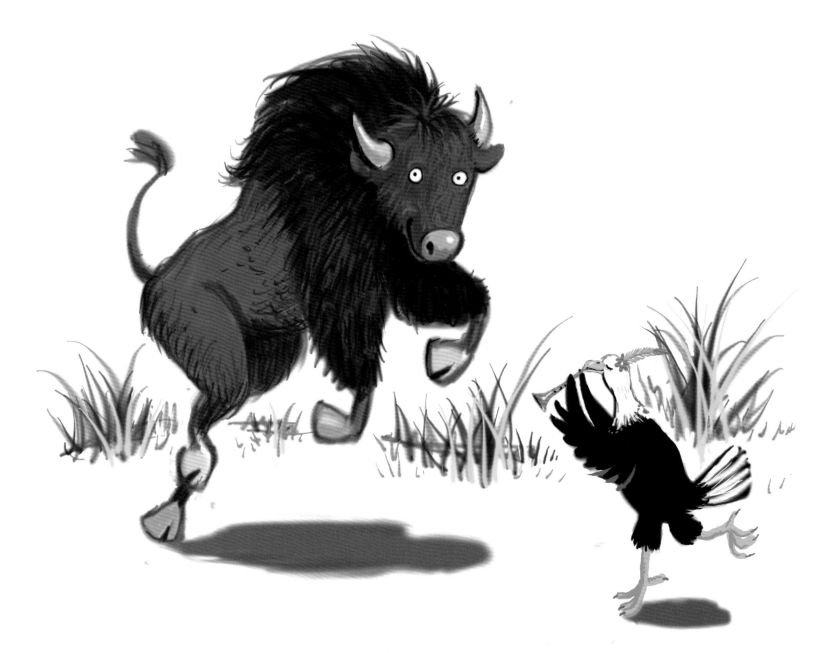

Ray the buffalo now knows what he needs to do each day.
He is excited because he will dance and play as Emily shows the way.

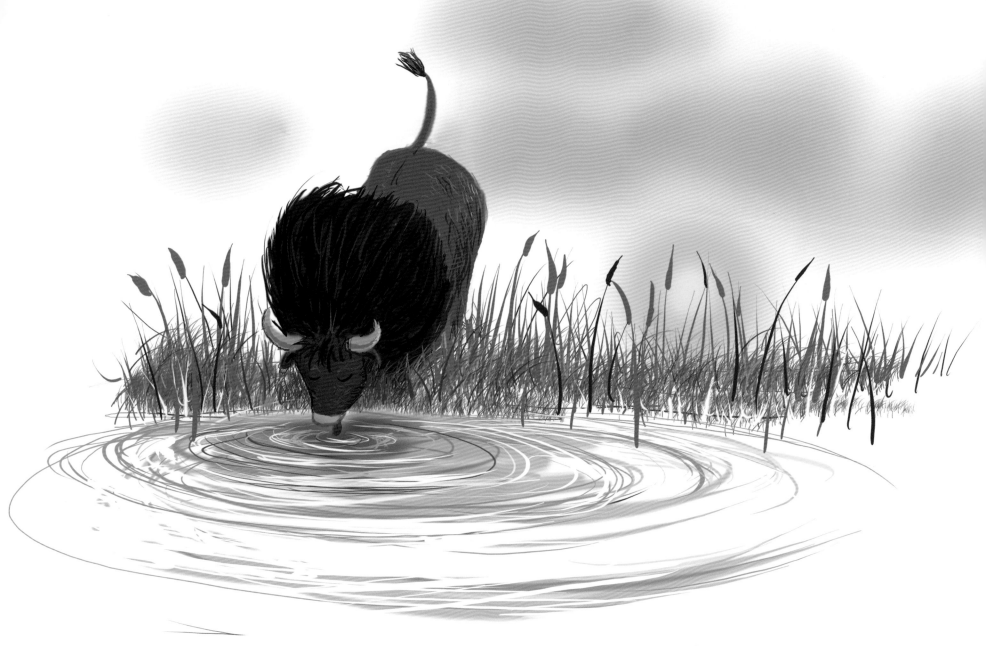

Ray the buffalo drinks his water to stay healthy and strong
at the beginning of a new day's dawn.

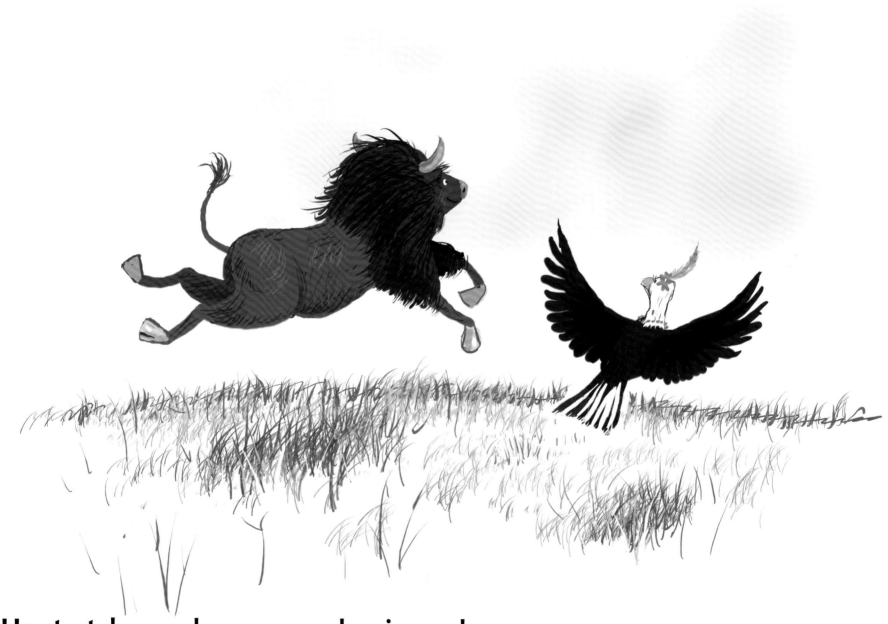

He stretches and prances as he sings a happy song.
Ray now moves fast and now dances along.

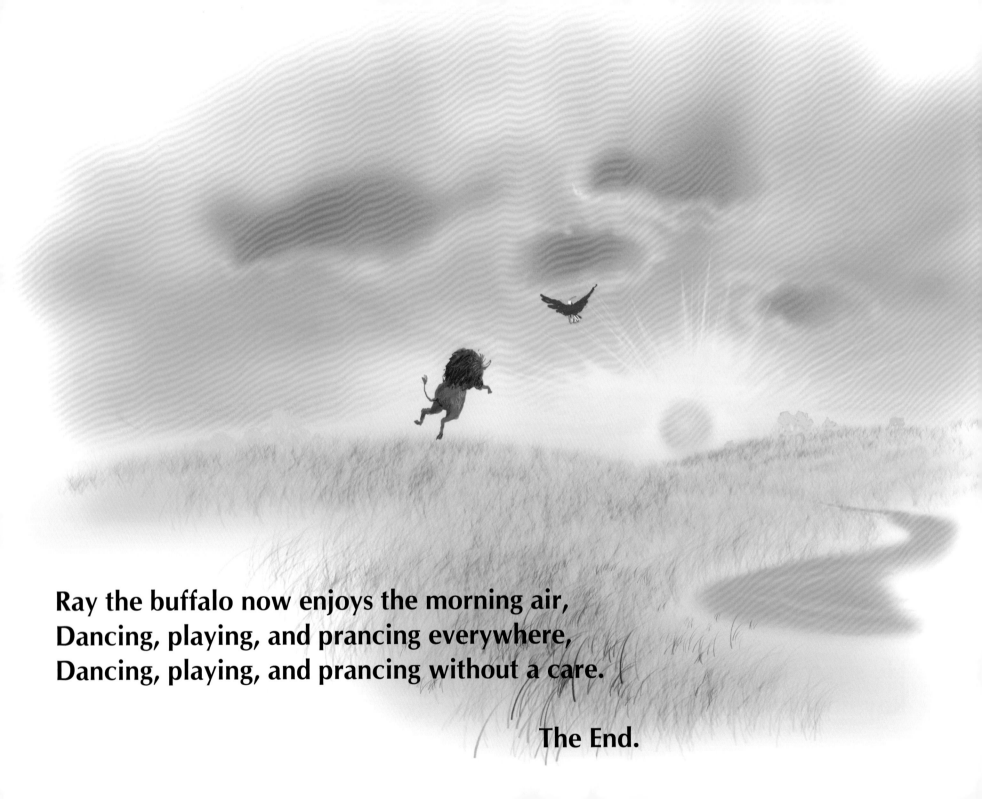

Ray the buffalo now enjoys the morning air,
Dancing, playing, and prancing everywhere,
Dancing, playing, and prancing without a care.

The End.

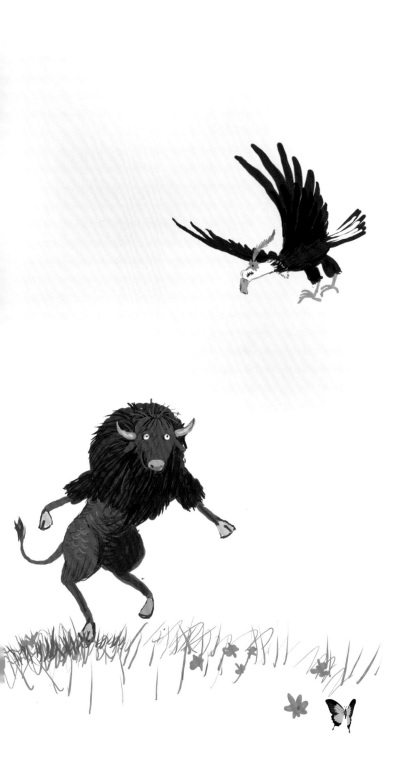

RAY THE BUFFALO "CHAT TIME"

Ray the buffalo and Emily the eagle
wants you to get moving and find your talents.

The buffalo, though appearing slow,
can run very fast and can leap great heights.

The eagle, though small, has great strength and can soar.

Discover your new found strengths,
as Ray the buffalo has, and soar like Emily the eagle!

Ray has questions for you:

- Will you do your best?
- Will you stay healthy and strong?
- Will you have the energy to be ready to go?

Emily has questions for you, too:

- Will you soar?
- Will you get moving?
- Will you stay healthy and strong?

MEET THE AUTHOR AND ILLUSTRATOR

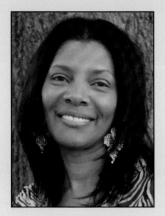

WILHEIMINA LONG

Wilheimina Long is a graphic designer/fine artist specializing in painting and line drawings. She received her B.A. degree in Fine Arts from the University of Mary Washington where she met Ron Miller, the illustrator, as she was a college intern under his direction at his Black Cat Studio. Now many years later, they team as author and illustrator in the development of her first children's book. She is an advocate for children, where she founded in 1999 the non-profit, Youth Matter Inc. Creating what is to become the Ray book series is so very dear to her heart, as her desire is to motivate and encourage children to be their best and to always strive to excel. She also continues to work toward her entrepreneur goals.

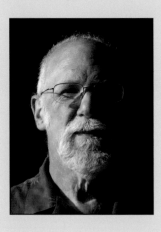

RON MILLER

Ron Miller is an illustrator/author specializing in science, astronomy, science fiction and fantasy. In addition to providing artwork for many magazine and book publishers, his special interest is in exciting young people about science and in recent years has focused on writing books for young adults. To date he has more than fifty titles to his credit. He has also designed postage stamps and worked on motion pictures as a production designer and special effects artist. You can visit him online at www.black-cat-studios.com.

To purchase "The Story of Ray the Buffalo", Ray and Emily buttons, stickers, and other items visit the online store at:

www.raythebuffalo.com

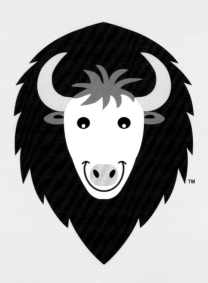

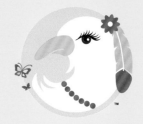

JELLYBEANS
Children's Books

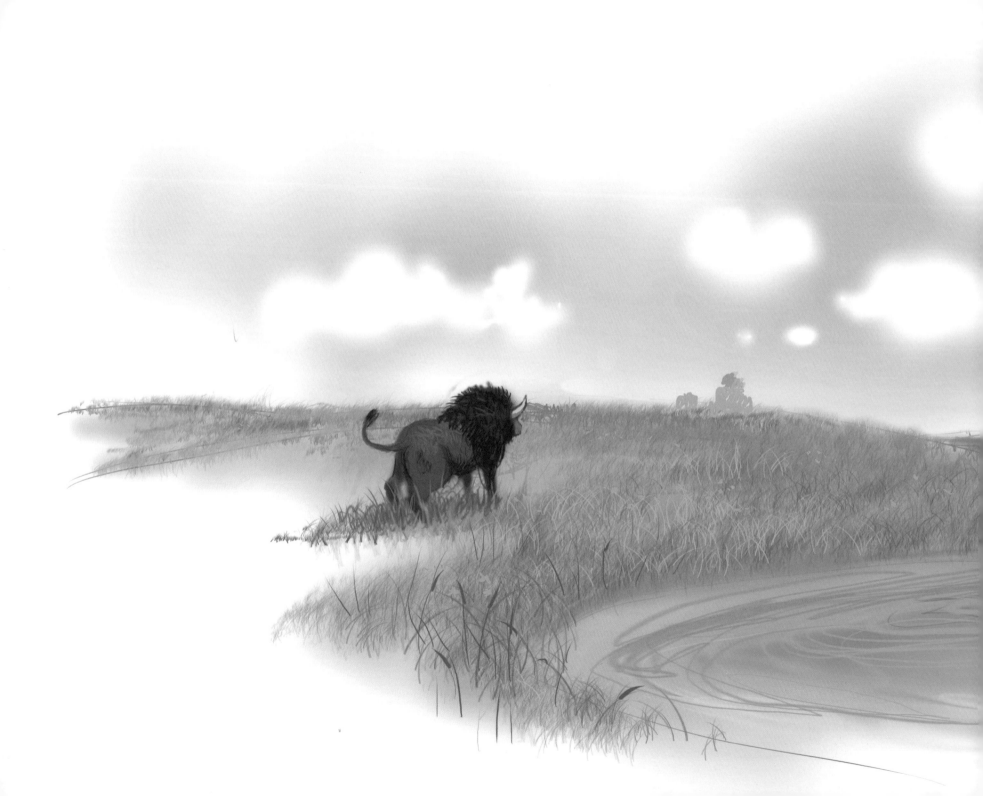